Barrett's Esophagus

Coping with Pre-Cancerous Esophageal Changes and Promoting Digestive Health

Early Detection, Symptom Control, GERD Management, Preventive Care, Reducing Cancer Risk and Lifestyle Strategies for Esophageal Health

Graham Julian Oliver

Disclaimer

The information provided in this book, *Barrett's Esophagus - Coping with Pre-Cancerous Esophageal Changes and Promoting Digestive Health*, is intended for educational and informational purposes only. It is not a substitute for professional medical advice, diagnosis, or treatment. Always seek the advice of your physician or other qualified health provider with any questions you may have regarding a medical condition or treatment. Never disregard professional medical advice or delay in seeking it because of something you have read in this book.

The author and publisher do not endorse any specific individual, product, website, organization, or other names that may be referenced or mentioned within this book. The content is provided solely for informational purposes, and the author and publisher are not responsible for any consequences arising from the use of this information.

Individual experiences may vary, and the information presented here may not be suitable for everyone. Always consult with a healthcare professional before making any changes to your health regimen or lifestyle.

By reading this book, you acknowledge and agree that you are using this information at your own risk, and you will not hold the author or publisher liable for any damages or issues that may arise from its use.

About This Book

Barrett's Esophagus - Coping with Pre-Cancerous Esophageal Changes and Promoting Digestive Health: Early Detection, Symptom Control, GERD Management, Preventive Care, Reducing Cancer Risk, and Lifestyle Strategies for Esophageal Health is an essential resource for individuals navigating the complexities of Barrett's Esophagus. This comprehensive guide delves into critical aspects of understanding, diagnosing, and managing this condition, while emphasizing the importance of preventive care and lifestyle adjustments to promote overall esophageal and digestive health.

Understanding Barrett's Esophagus is key to managing the condition effectively. This book begins by offering a thorough exploration of what Barrett's Esophagus is, its connection to GERD, and the pre-cancerous risks associated with the condition. Highlighting the importance of early diagnosis, readers gain insight into how recognizing and managing GERD—a major precursor—can prevent the progression to Barrett's. With a strong focus on esophageal care, the book educates readers about how lifestyle adjustments and diet impact the digestive system, providing practical advice for maintaining optimal esophageal health.

A significant portion of the book is dedicated to early detection and diagnosis of Barrett's Esophagus. By recognizing the early symptoms and understanding the role of acid reflux, readers are better equipped to take proactive steps toward diagnosis. The use of endoscopy, biopsy, and routine check-ups are outlined as vital tools in identifying and monitoring the condition. The inclusion of family medical history and understanding individual risk factors also plays a critical role in ensuring accurate and early diagnosis, reducing the chances of misdiagnosis.

Managing GERD is pivotal in preventing the development of Barrett's Esophagus, and this book provides an in-depth look at GERD management strategies. From medication options like PPIs and H2 blockers to crucial lifestyle changes such as dietary adjustments, avoiding trigger foods, and stress management, readers learn how to alleviate chronic acid reflux and prevent further esophageal damage. The importance of weight management, smoking cessation, and reducing alcohol intake is also highlighted, providing a holistic approach to managing GERD and preventing Barrett's Esophagus.

Symptom control and lifestyle modifications are essential for individuals living with Barrett's Esophagus. This book empowers readers to identify their symptom triggers and offers practical advice on adjusting meal portions, timings, and positions for sleeping to minimize reflux. Stress management is also explored in depth, offering simple techniques to alleviate stress-related symptoms. Additionally, the importance of hydration, food allergies, and daily exercise is emphasized as part of a comprehensive approach to improving esophageal health and controlling symptoms.

Preventive care is central to managing Barrett's Esophagus, and this book emphasizes the necessity of regular medical monitoring and proactive health management. Through routine endoscopic surveillance and tracking of cellular changes, individuals can prevent the progression of Barrett's Esophagus and avoid further esophageal damage. The book highlights the role of PPIs and other long-term medication management strategies, alongside the importance of seeking early intervention for new or worsening symptoms. By encouraging preventive care, the book equips readers to take charge of their health and reduce the risks associated with Barrett's.

The risk of esophageal cancer is a major concern for individuals with Barrett's Esophagus, and this book thoroughly addresses ways to reduce this risk. Lifestyle changes such as smoking cessation, managing alcohol consumption, and adopting a plant-based diet rich in antioxidants and fiber are emphasized as key factors in cancer prevention. Regular monitoring for dysplasia and the use of medications or surgical interventions when necessary are discussed in detail, ensuring that readers understand the importance of early detection and proactive treatment in reducing cancer risk.

Dietary changes play a crucial role in promoting esophageal health, and this book provides clear guidance on the best and worst foods for individuals with Barrett's Esophagus. The importance of a balanced, anti-inflammatory diet is highlighted, with practical tips for avoiding acidic foods and beverages, incorporating fiber-rich foods, and preparing reflux-friendly meals. The book also emphasizes the benefits of smaller, more frequent meals and staying hydrated to support overall digestive health.

Medical treatments for Barrett's Esophagus are explained in an accessible yet informative manner. The role of proton pump inhibitors, H2 blockers, and over-the-counter antacids in managing acid suppression is detailed, while more advanced treatments like radiofrequency ablation and photodynamic therapy are discussed as options for treating dysplasia. The pros and cons of long-term medication use are also examined, providing readers with a well-rounded understanding of their treatment options.

For individuals who may require surgery, the book offers an insightful overview of surgical interventions such as Nissen fundoplication and esophagectomy.

Readers are guided through what to expect during recovery and the dietary care needed post-surgery. The book also outlines the risks and benefits of minimally invasive surgeries, offering a balanced perspective on when surgery may be necessary and how to choose the right specialist.

Common concerns and frequently asked questions are addressed to provide clarity and reassurance to those managing Barrett's Esophagus. From understanding the possibility of cancer development to navigating long-term medication needs, the book provides thoughtful answers to key concerns.

This book is an indispensable guide for individuals seeking to understand and manage Barrett's Esophagus. It offers expert insights into early detection, symptom control, GERD management, and preventive care, while also providing practical lifestyle strategies for promoting esophageal health and reducing the risk of esophageal cancer. With its clear and engaging tone, this book serves as a valuable resource for anyone looking to take a proactive approach to their esophageal health.

Table of Contents

Introduction:

What is Barrett's Esophagus?

Barrett's Esophagus is a condition where the tissue lining the esophagus changes to tissue that resembles the lining of the intestine. This transformation occurs due to prolonged exposure to stomach acid, which damages the esophageal lining. These changes are typically a response to chronic acid reflux or gastroesophageal reflux disease (GERD), and they can increase the risk of developing esophageal cancer.

Patients with Barrett's Esophagus usually do not notice symptoms themselves, as the condition is often silent. It is typically detected during an endoscopy. The primary concern with Barrett's Esophagus is that the altered cells can become dysplastic (precancerous), which is why regular monitoring is essential.

Why Does Barrett's Esophagus Occur?

Barrett's Esophagus occurs when long-term acid reflux causes damage to the esophageal lining. Chronic inflammation leads to the replacement of normal squamous cells with intestinal-like cells, known as metaplasia. Risk factors include GERD, smoking, obesity, and male gender, particularly in middle-aged individuals.

To reduce the likelihood of Barrett's Esophagus, managing acid reflux through dietary changes, medications like proton pump inhibitors (PPIs), and weight management is crucial. Early detection through screening in individuals with persistent GERD symptoms can prevent further complications.

How Barrett's Relates to GERD (Gastroesophageal Reflux Disease)

Barrett's Esophagus is strongly linked to GERD, a condition where stomach acid flows backward into the esophagus, irritating the lining. GERD symptoms, like heartburn and acid regurgitation, when untreated, can lead to chronic inflammation, eventually causing the cellular changes that define Barrett's Esophagus.

Preventing Barrett's Esophagus often starts with managing GERD effectively. This can include using acid-reducing medications, adopting a reflux-friendly diet (e.g., avoiding spicy or fatty foods), and making lifestyle changes such as elevating the head of the bed and not eating before bedtime.

Pre-cancerous Implications: What it Means

Barrett's Esophagus is considered a pre-cancerous condition because the cellular changes in the esophagus can lead to esophageal adenocarcinoma, a serious form of cancer. While the risk is relatively low (less than 1% per year), the progression from metaplasia to dysplasia, and then to cancer, requires vigilant monitoring.

Regular endoscopies with biopsies are recommended for patients diagnosed with Barrett's Esophagus. If dysplasia is detected, treatments such as radiofrequency ablation (RFA) or endoscopic resection may be employed to remove or destroy abnormal cells before they become cancerous.

Importance of Early Diagnosis

Early diagnosis of Barrett's Esophagus is critical because it allows for timely intervention and reduces the risk of developing esophageal cancer. Screening is often recommended for individuals with long-term GERD, especially those with additional risk factors such as smoking or obesity.

Once diagnosed, patients should follow a structured surveillance plan with their healthcare provider. This typically involves routine endoscopies to monitor for dysplasia, coupled with lifestyle and dietary modifications to control GERD and prevent further esophageal damage.

Digestive Health and Esophageal Care

The Role of the Esophagus in Digestion

The esophagus is a muscular tube that transports food and liquids from the mouth to the stomach, playing a crucial role in digestion. As you swallow, the muscles of the esophagus contract in a wave-like motion called peristalsis, pushing food downward into the stomach for further digestion. This process is vital to ensure that nutrients are absorbed properly in the digestive tract.

However, any malfunction in the esophagus can disrupt this process. Conditions such as GERD (gastroesophageal reflux disease) or Barrett's Esophagus can damage the esophagus, leading to discomfort and poor digestion. Ensuring the esophagus functions properly is key to maintaining overall digestive health.

Key Factors Affecting Esophageal Health

Several factors impact esophageal health, including diet, stress, and the frequency of acid reflux. GERD, for example, causes stomach acid to back up into the esophagus, irritating the lining and potentially leading to Barrett's Esophagus, a pre-cancerous condition. Smoking, excessive alcohol consumption, and obesity are also significant contributors to esophageal damage.

To protect the esophagus, it's essential to avoid trigger foods (like spicy or acidic items), quit smoking, and manage weight through regular exercise. Paying attention to the body's signals, such as persistent heartburn or difficulty swallowing, can help prevent long-term damage.

Diet's Impact on Esophageal and Digestive Health

A balanced diet plays a major role in maintaining the health of both the esophagus and the digestive system.

Foods rich in fiber, fruits, vegetables, lean proteins, and whole grains promote digestion and minimize acid reflux. Avoiding trigger foods like caffeine, alcohol, fatty or fried foods, and acidic beverages helps reduce irritation to the esophageal lining.

Incorporating smaller, more frequent meals instead of large ones can also reduce pressure on the lower esophageal sphincter (LES), minimizing reflux. It's crucial to stay hydrated and consume adequate fiber to promote smooth digestion, preventing constipation and reducing strain on the esophagus.

Importance of Lifestyle Adjustments

Lifestyle changes are critical for maintaining esophageal health and preventing conditions like GERD or Barrett's Esophagus. Quitting smoking, reducing alcohol consumption, and maintaining a healthy weight can significantly decrease the risk of acid reflux. Elevating the head during sleep and avoiding lying down immediately after eating also help prevent acid from flowing back into the esophagus.

Incorporating stress-reducing practices like yoga, meditation, or deep breathing exercises can also improve digestive health. Stress has been shown to exacerbate digestive issues, so managing it is essential for a healthy esophagus and overall digestive function.

How to Maintain a Healthy Digestive System

Maintaining a healthy digestive system involves a combination of proper nutrition, hydration, exercise, and regular medical check-ups. Eating a well-balanced diet with plenty of fiber, fruits, and vegetables helps promote healthy digestion and reduce the risk of constipation and acid reflux. Staying hydrated is equally important, as it helps break down food and absorb nutrients effectively.

In addition to diet, regular physical activity stimulates the muscles in the digestive tract, promoting efficient digestion.

CHAPTER 1:

Early Detection and Diagnosis of Barrett's Esophagus

Recognizing Early Symptoms

Early symptoms of Barrett's esophagus can often mirror those of gastroesophageal reflux disease (GERD), making it essential to identify and monitor them closely. Common symptoms include persistent heartburn, difficulty swallowing, and regurgitation of food or sour liquid. Keeping a symptom diary can be beneficial; note when symptoms occur, their severity, and potential triggers to discuss with your healthcare provider.

It's crucial to pay attention to any changes in symptoms or the emergence of new ones. For instance, if heartburn worsens or becomes more frequent despite treatment, it may signal progression. Consulting with a healthcare professional for proper evaluation and guidance can lead to timely interventions and better management of symptoms.

Understanding Acid Reflux and Its Role

Acid reflux occurs when stomach acid flows back into the esophagus, causing irritation and inflammation. This condition is often linked to lifestyle factors such as diet, obesity, and smoking, which can exacerbate symptoms. Understanding the triggers of acid reflux is vital for managing symptoms effectively. Keeping a food diary and avoiding known irritants, like spicy foods, caffeine, and alcohol, can help mitigate reflux episodes.

Incorporating lifestyle changes can significantly reduce acid reflux symptoms. Eating smaller, more frequent meals, maintaining a healthy weight, and elevating the head of your bed can improve digestion and minimize reflux events. If symptoms persist, discussing potential medications with your healthcare provider can help manage acid levels and protect the esophagus.

Diagnosing GERD: A Precursor to Barrett's

Diagnosing GERD is the first step in preventing Barrett's esophagus. A healthcare provider will typically evaluate your symptoms, medical history, and any lifestyle factors that contribute to reflux. They may also perform a physical examination. To confirm the diagnosis, a doctor may recommend additional tests, such as a pH probe study to measure acid levels in the esophagus over a 24-hour period.

Proper diagnosis is essential for effective management and can include medications, lifestyle modifications, and monitoring of symptoms. If left untreated, GERD can lead to complications, including Barrett's esophagus. Regular follow-ups and adjustments to your management plan can help control symptoms and prevent further complications.

Endoscopy: The Gold Standard for Diagnosis

An upper endoscopy is a procedure that allows doctors to visualize the esophagus and stomach. It involves inserting a thin, flexible tube with a camera into the mouth and down the throat. This procedure is typically performed under sedation, making it comfortable for the patient. Endoscopy can help identify inflammation, strictures, and Barrett's esophagus, providing crucial information for further management.

Patients may need to prepare for an endoscopy by fasting for several hours prior to the procedure. After the endoscopy, it's common to experience a sore throat, but recovery is usually quick. Discuss any findings with your healthcare provider, who will outline the next steps based on the results.

Biopsy Procedures for Barrett's Detection

During an endoscopy, a biopsy can be performed to obtain small samples of tissue from the esophagus. This procedure involves using specialized tools to take tissue samples, which are then sent to a laboratory for analysis. Biopsies are critical for confirming Barrett's esophagus, as they help identify abnormal cell changes that may lead to cancer.

Preparation for a biopsy is similar to that of an endoscopy. After the procedure, you may experience mild discomfort or throat soreness, which typically resolves quickly. Your doctor will discuss the results and any necessary follow-up actions based on the biopsy findings.

Importance of Routine Check-ups

Routine check-ups are essential for early detection and management of Barrett's esophagus. Regular visits to a healthcare provider can help monitor symptoms and the progression of GERD. During these appointments, discussing any changes in symptoms or new concerns is vital to ensure timely intervention.

Additionally, your healthcare provider may recommend regular endoscopies for those with a history of GERD or Barrett's esophagus. Following the recommended schedule for check-ups can lead to early identification of potential complications, allowing for prompt treatment and improved outcomes.

Blood Tests and Imaging for Related Conditions

Blood tests and imaging studies can provide additional insights into esophageal health and related conditions. Blood tests can help identify potential deficiencies or underlying health issues that may affect digestion, while imaging studies like X-rays or CT scans can assess the esophagus and surrounding organs for abnormalities.

Your healthcare provider will determine the appropriate tests based on your symptoms and medical history. Following through with these tests can enhance understanding of your overall health and help in developing a comprehensive management plan.

Discussing Family History with Your Doctor

Understanding your family history is vital in assessing the risk of Barrett's esophagus and related conditions. Discussing any family history of esophageal cancer or GERD with your doctor allows them to evaluate your risk factors more accurately. This information can inform decisions regarding screening and preventive measures.

Be proactive in communicating family medical history during consultations. If you have a significant family history of these conditions, your healthcare provider may recommend earlier or more frequent screenings to monitor for changes and address any concerns effectively.

Screening Recommendations for High-Risk Individuals

High-risk individuals, such as those with chronic GERD or a family history of esophageal cancer, should follow specific screening recommendations. Guidelines often suggest regular endoscopies to monitor the esophagus for changes associated with Barrett's esophagus. Your doctor can tailor a screening schedule based on your individual risk factors.

Adhering to these recommendations is crucial for early detection and intervention. By proactively participating in your healthcare plan, you can significantly reduce the risk of complications and improve long-term health outcomes.

The Role of Medical History in Diagnosis

A thorough medical history plays a critical role in diagnosing Barrett's esophagus and related conditions. Your healthcare provider will ask detailed questions about your symptoms, previous medical issues, and family history. This information helps them assess your risk factors and determine the appropriate diagnostic tests.

Providing accurate and comprehensive information during your consultations enhances the diagnostic process. Being honest about your symptoms, lifestyle, and any medications you're taking can significantly impact your healthcare provider's understanding and treatment recommendations.

Differentiating Barrett's from Other Esophageal Issues

Differentiating Barrett's esophagus from other esophageal issues is essential for appropriate management. Symptoms like heartburn, difficulty swallowing, and chest pain can overlap with various conditions. Your healthcare provider will use a combination of medical history, physical examinations, and diagnostic tests to distinguish Barrett's from other potential causes.

If diagnosed with Barrett's esophagus, understanding the specific nature of your condition is vital. This knowledge can help you engage in informed discussions with your healthcare provider about treatment options, lifestyle modifications, and necessary monitoring.

Misdiagnosis Risks: How to Avoid Them

Misdiagnosis can occur when symptoms of Barrett's esophagus overlap with other conditions, leading to inappropriate treatment. To minimize this risk, ensure that you communicate openly with your healthcare provider about all your symptoms, their frequency, and any relevant medical history. Providing a complete picture will help them make a more accurate diagnosis.

Additionally, seeking a second opinion or consulting a specialist when unsure about a diagnosis can provide further clarity. Being proactive and engaged in your healthcare can lead to timely and appropriate treatment, improving your overall health outcomes.

When to Seek a Specialist's Opinion

Knowing when to seek a specialist's opinion can be crucial for effective management of Barrett's esophagus. If you experience persistent symptoms despite treatment, or if new symptoms arise, consulting a gastroenterologist is advisable. These specialists can offer advanced diagnostic tools and targeted treatment options.

Establishing a relationship with a specialist ensures access to comprehensive care tailored to your specific needs. They can guide you through the complexities of your condition, including lifestyle changes, medical treatments, and the importance of ongoing monitoring.

CHAPTER 2:

Managing GERD to Prevent Barrett's Esophagus

The Link between GERD and Barrett's Esophagus

Gastroesophageal reflux disease (GERD) is a chronic condition characterized by the backflow of stomach acid into the esophagus, leading to inflammation and damage. Over time, this persistent acid exposure can result in changes to the esophageal lining, a condition known as Barrett's esophagus, which increases the risk of esophageal cancer. Understanding this link emphasizes the need for early intervention in managing GERD to prevent progression to more serious conditions.

To mitigate the risk of Barrett's esophagus, it is essential to recognize and manage GERD symptoms promptly. Regular check-ups with a healthcare provider can help monitor esophageal health and address any changes early on. Staying informed about the potential risks associated with untreated GERD can motivate individuals to adhere to treatment plans and lifestyle modifications aimed at promoting esophageal health.

Common Symptoms of GERD

GERD presents with a variety of symptoms that can significantly impact daily life. The most common include heartburn, a burning sensation in the chest; regurgitation, where sour or bitter acid backs up into the throat or mouth; and difficulty swallowing. These symptoms may occur after meals or when lying down, indicating a need for prompt evaluation and management.

If you suspect you have GERD, keeping a symptom diary can be helpful. Record when symptoms occur, their intensity, and any potential triggers. This information can be valuable for healthcare providers in diagnosing and tailoring an effective treatment plan to manage symptoms and improve quality of life.

Importance of Treating Chronic Acid Reflux

Treating chronic acid reflux is crucial to prevent complications, including esophageal damage and Barrett's esophagus. Untreated GERD can lead to inflammation, ulcers, and narrowing of the esophagus, which can make swallowing difficult. Furthermore, long-term exposure to stomach acid significantly increases the risk of developing esophageal cancer.

To effectively manage chronic acid reflux, a comprehensive approach is essential. This may include lifestyle changes, medication, and regular monitoring by healthcare professionals. Taking proactive steps to manage symptoms not only alleviates discomfort but also safeguards long-term health.

Medications for GERD: PPIs, H2 Blockers, and Antacids

Proton pump inhibitors (PPIs), H2 blockers, and antacids are commonly prescribed medications for managing GERD. PPIs, such as omeprazole, reduce stomach acid production, providing significant symptom relief. H2 blockers, like ranitidine, also decrease acid production but work differently and are generally milder. Antacids neutralize existing stomach acid and offer quick relief from heartburn.

Consulting a healthcare provider is essential to determine the most appropriate medication based on individual needs and severity of symptoms. It's crucial to follow prescribed dosages and schedules, and regularly review medication effectiveness with a doctor to ensure optimal management of GERD.

Dietary Changes to Manage GERD

Making dietary changes can significantly impact the management of GERD symptoms. Incorporating more fruits, vegetables, whole grains, and lean proteins can help promote digestive health. Foods rich in fiber can aid digestion, while smaller, more frequent meals can reduce pressure on the stomach, minimizing reflux episodes.

Avoiding overly spicy, fatty, or acidic foods is also key. Keeping a food journal can help identify personal triggers and facilitate adjustments to one's diet. By making conscious food choices, individuals can create a meal plan that supports esophageal health and minimizes GERD symptoms.

Avoiding Trigger Foods for Acid Reflux

Identifying and avoiding trigger foods is vital for effective GERD management. Common culprits include caffeine, chocolate, citrus fruits, tomatoes, garlic, onions, and carbonated beverages. These foods can exacerbate symptoms and lead to increased acid production or relaxation of the lower esophageal sphincter.

To effectively avoid triggers, consider an elimination diet where suspected foods are removed for a period and then gradually reintroduced to assess their impact. This process can help pinpoint specific triggers, enabling individuals to make informed dietary choices that align with their health needs.

Elevating the Head While Sleeping

Elevating the head while sleeping is an effective strategy to reduce nighttime GERD symptoms. This position helps prevent stomach acid from flowing back into the esophagus, reducing the likelihood of nighttime heartburn and discomfort. Using a wedge pillow or raising the head of the bed by 6 to 8 inches can make a significant difference in symptom control.

When adjusting your sleeping environment, ensure the elevation is comfortable and maintains proper spinal alignment. Experimenting with different angles may help identify the most effective position for minimizing reflux during sleep.

Stress Management Techniques for GERD

Stress can exacerbate GERD symptoms, making stress management an essential part of treatment. Techniques such as mindfulness meditation, yoga, deep breathing exercises, and regular physical activity can help reduce stress levels and improve overall well-being. Engaging in enjoyable activities and hobbies can also provide necessary mental breaks.

Incorporating stress-reducing practices into your daily routine can enhance your ability to cope with GERD. Setting aside time for relaxation and self-care can improve not only mental health but also contribute to better digestive health.

Weight Loss and Its Impact on GERD

Excess weight can increase pressure on the stomach, pushing acid into the esophagus and worsening GERD symptoms. Weight loss can significantly alleviate these pressures and reduce the frequency and severity of reflux episodes. Even a modest weight loss of 5-10% can lead to noticeable improvements in symptoms for many individuals.

To achieve and maintain a healthy weight, focus on balanced nutrition and regular physical activity.

Consulting with a healthcare provider or a registered dietitian can provide personalized guidance and support for developing a sustainable weight loss plan tailored to your needs.

Timing of Meals and Its Effect on Reflux

Meal timing plays a crucial role in managing GERD symptoms. Eating large meals or consuming food too close to bedtime can increase the risk of reflux. It's advisable to eat smaller, more frequent meals and to finish eating at least two to three hours before lying down or going to bed.

Planning meals ahead of time can facilitate better timing and portion control. Establishing a routine can help regulate digestive patterns and minimize discomfort associated with GERD.

Smoking Cessation for GERD Control

Smoking is a significant risk factor for GERD, as it can weaken the lower esophageal sphincter and increase acid production. Quitting smoking can lead to substantial improvements in GERD symptoms and overall digestive health. Many resources are available, including support groups, counseling, and nicotine replacement therapies, to assist individuals in their cessation efforts.

Creating a quit plan that outlines personal motivations, triggers, and support systems can enhance the likelihood of success. Tracking progress and celebrating milestones can provide additional motivation and reinforce the commitment to quit smoking.

Reducing Alcohol Consumption

Alcohol can relax the lower esophageal sphincter and increase stomach acid production, contributing to GERD symptoms. Reducing alcohol intake can improve symptom control and promote overall digestive health. It's advisable to limit alcohol consumption to moderate levels, which is typically defined as up to one drink per day for women and two for men.

Setting personal goals for alcohol consumption can help in managing intake. Exploring non-alcoholic alternatives and engaging in social activities that do not revolve around drinking can facilitate healthier habits and support better GERD management.

Regular Follow-Ups with a Gastroenterologist

Regular follow-ups with a gastroenterologist are crucial for managing GERD and monitoring for potential complications like Barrett's esophagus. These appointments provide an opportunity to discuss symptom control, medication effectiveness, and any necessary adjustments to treatment plans. It's important to communicate openly about changes in symptoms or any new concerns that arise.

Scheduling these follow-ups and preparing questions or topics to discuss can help maximize the benefits of each appointment. By maintaining an ongoing relationship with a gastroenterologist, individuals can receive tailored care that adapts to their evolving health needs.

CHAPTER 3:

Symptom Control and Lifestyle Modifications

Identifying Key Symptom Triggers

To manage Barrett's esophagus effectively, it's crucial to identify what triggers your symptoms. Common triggers include spicy foods, acidic foods like tomatoes and citrus, and large meals. Keeping a food diary can help you pinpoint these triggers by noting what you eat and how it affects your symptoms.

Once you've identified your triggers, you can begin to modify your diet accordingly. For instance, if you notice that spicy dishes lead to discomfort, consider substituting them with milder options. This tailored approach to your diet will help you minimize flare-ups and maintain better control over your symptoms.

Modifying Meal Portions and Timings

Adjusting meal portions and timings can significantly alleviate esophageal discomfort. Eating smaller, more frequent meals instead of large ones can help reduce the pressure on the esophageal sphincter, minimizing the risk of reflux. Aim for five to six small meals throughout the day rather than two or three large ones.

Additionally, try to eat your last meal at least two to three hours before bedtime. This allows your stomach to digest food properly and reduces the chances of acid reflux while you sleep. Practicing mindful eating, such as eating slowly and without distractions, can further enhance digestion and help you recognize when you're full.

Best Positions for Sleep to Reduce Reflux

The position in which you sleep can impact the severity of reflux symptoms. Elevating your head while sleeping, either with a wedge pillow or by adjusting the bed frame, can help keep stomach acid from rising into the esophagus. Aim for an elevation of about 30 degrees to effectively minimize nighttime reflux.

Avoid sleeping on your back, as this position can exacerbate symptoms. Instead, consider sleeping on your left side. This position can help reduce acid reflux symptoms, as it allows for better digestion and less pressure on the stomach.

Maintaining a Healthy Weight

Maintaining a healthy weight is essential for managing Barrett's esophagus. Excess weight can increase abdominal pressure, which may lead to a higher risk of reflux symptoms. If you are overweight, consider making gradual lifestyle changes, such as incorporating healthier foods and regular physical activity to achieve a balanced weight.

Aim for a balanced diet rich in whole grains, lean proteins, fruits, and vegetables while limiting processed foods high in sugar and fat. Regular exercise, such as walking, swimming, or cycling, can not only help with weight loss but also enhance overall digestive health and reduce stress.

How Stress Aggravates Symptoms

Stress can significantly worsen the symptoms of Barrett's esophagus. It triggers the release of hormones that may increase stomach acid production, leading to increased reflux. Recognizing stressors in your life and understanding their impact on your symptoms can empower you to manage them better.

Finding effective ways to cope with stress is crucial. Incorporating relaxation techniques such as mindfulness, meditation, or yoga can help lower stress levels. By making these techniques a part of your daily routine, you may find an improvement in your overall digestive health and symptom control.

Simple Stress-Relief Techniques

To combat stress, implement simple yet effective techniques into your daily routine. Deep breathing exercises can be practiced anytime, helping to calm the mind and body. For instance, take a moment to inhale deeply through your nose, hold for a few seconds, and then exhale slowly through your mouth.

Engaging in physical activity, even a short walk, can help release endorphins, improving your mood and reducing stress. Activities like journaling, listening to music, or spending time in nature can also serve as excellent outlets for stress relief.

Understanding Food Allergies and Intolerances

Understanding food allergies and intolerances is key to managing Barrett's esophagus. Keep an eye on how specific foods affect your symptoms and consult with a healthcare provider to discuss potential food allergies. This process often involves elimination diets or allergy testing to identify problematic foods.

If you suspect certain foods are causing issues, consider keeping a detailed food diary to track your intake and symptoms. Once identified, you can avoid these foods and explore alternatives that are less likely to trigger your reflux.

Importance of Hydration for Esophageal Health

Staying hydrated is vital for overall digestive health, including esophageal well-being. Water helps neutralize stomach acid and aids digestion. Aim to drink at least eight 8-ounce glasses of water daily, adjusting based on your individual needs and activity level.

Incorporate water-rich foods like fruits and vegetables into your diet. If you struggle with hydration, consider carrying a water bottle with you throughout the day as a reminder to drink regularly. Avoid carbonated beverages, as they can increase bloating and exacerbate symptoms.

Avoiding Tight Clothing Around the Abdomen

Wearing tight clothing around the abdomen can increase pressure on the stomach, contributing to reflux symptoms. Opt for looser-fitting clothes that allow for comfortable movement. Avoiding belts or waistbands that dig into your stomach can also help minimize discomfort.

Choosing clothing made from breathable fabrics can enhance comfort and help maintain a healthy digestive system. If you notice that certain outfits trigger your symptoms, consider changing your wardrobe to prioritize comfort over style.

Reducing Caffeine Intake for Symptom Control

Caffeine can exacerbate reflux symptoms by relaxing the lower esophageal sphincter. Reducing or eliminating caffeinated beverages, such as coffee, tea, and soda, can help control symptoms. Consider substituting with herbal teas or decaffeinated options, which may be gentler on your stomach.

When making changes to your caffeine intake, do so gradually to prevent withdrawal symptoms. Pay attention to how your body responds and adjust accordingly, keeping track of your symptoms in a food journal for better insight.

Importance of Chewing Food Thoroughly

Thoroughly chewing your food aids in digestion and can reduce the risk of reflux. Breaking food down into smaller pieces allows enzymes in your saliva to begin the digestive process, making it easier for your stomach to do its job. Aim to chew each bite 20 to 30 times before swallowing.

Taking time to chew food thoroughly also encourages mindful eating, which can help prevent overeating. By being present during meals and focusing on the flavors and textures, you can enhance your overall eating experience and promote better digestion.

Benefits of Regular Light Exercise

Incorporating regular light exercise into your routine can be beneficial for managing Barrett's esophagus. Activities like walking, swimming, or cycling improve circulation and help maintain a healthy weight, both of which can reduce reflux symptoms. Aim for at least 30 minutes of moderate exercise most days of the week.

Start gradually if you're not used to exercising. Even short bursts of activity throughout the day can be beneficial. Consistency is key, so find activities you enjoy, making it easier to stick to your exercise routine and improve your overall digestive health.

Tracking Symptoms in a Daily Journal

Keeping a daily journal to track your symptoms can provide valuable insights into your condition. Note what you eat, your activities, and any symptoms you experience, including their intensity and duration. This practice can help you identify patterns and correlations between your diet, lifestyle, and symptom flare-ups.

Reviewing your journal regularly can guide your decisions about diet and lifestyle adjustments.

CHAPTER 4:

Preventive Care and Monitoring

Why Preventive Care is Crucial in Barrett's Esophagus

Preventive care is essential in Barrett's Esophagus (BE) because it helps manage the risk of progression to esophageal cancer. Regular medical oversight can detect changes early, allowing for timely interventions that can significantly reduce cancer risk. Individuals with BE should prioritize understanding their condition and work closely with their healthcare team to develop an effective management plan.

Engaging in preventive care also involves lifestyle changes that support digestive health. Eating a balanced diet, maintaining a healthy weight, and avoiding smoking can all contribute to reducing the risk of further complications associated with BE. Being informed and proactive about health can empower patients to take charge of their well-being.

Frequency of Medical Check-Ups

Regular medical check-ups are vital for individuals with Barrett's Esophagus to monitor their condition effectively. Patients should consult with their healthcare providers about the recommended frequency of visits, typically every six months to a year, depending on their specific risk factors and symptoms. These check-ups can help catch any changes early, allowing for adjustments in treatment or lifestyle as necessary.

During these visits, healthcare professionals can perform necessary evaluations and provide guidance on managing symptoms. Patients should be prepared to discuss any new or worsening symptoms, which can help tailor their treatment plan and ensure that they receive appropriate care.

Monitoring Symptom Changes

Monitoring symptom changes is crucial for individuals with Barrett's Esophagus as it allows for timely identification of any complications or progression of the condition. Patients should keep a detailed journal of their symptoms, including frequency, intensity, and any triggers they may identify. This log can be shared with healthcare providers during check-ups, facilitating informed discussions about necessary adjustments to treatment or lifestyle changes.

Patients should be vigilant for specific symptoms, such as difficulty swallowing, chest pain, or unexplained weight loss, and report these changes immediately. Early detection of symptom changes can lead to prompt medical intervention, potentially preventing serious complications related to Barrett's Esophagus.

Regular Endoscopic Surveillance

Regular endoscopic surveillance is a key component of managing Barrett's Esophagus, allowing for the direct observation of the esophageal lining. This procedure typically involves inserting a thin, flexible tube with a camera into the esophagus to identify any cellular changes that may indicate progression toward cancer. Depending on individual risk factors, surveillance may be recommended every 1 to 3 years.

Patients should prepare for endoscopy by following their healthcare provider's instructions regarding fasting and medication adjustments. This proactive approach ensures that any necessary interventions can be implemented promptly, helping to maintain esophageal health and reduce cancer risk.

Preventing Further Damage to the Esophagus

Preventing further damage to the esophagus involves a combination of lifestyle modifications and medical management. Patients should focus on avoiding foods and beverages that trigger acid reflux, such as spicy foods, citrus, caffeine, and alcohol. Eating smaller, more frequent meals can also help minimize pressure on the esophageal sphincter.

Additionally, patients should consider elevating the head of their bed to reduce nighttime reflux and avoid lying down immediately after eating. These strategies can help protect the esophagus from additional injury and promote overall digestive health.

Tracking Progression of Cellular Changes

Tracking the progression of cellular changes in Barrett's Esophagus is essential for determining the need for more aggressive treatment. Healthcare providers typically perform biopsies during endoscopic procedures to evaluate the cellular structure and identify dysplasia, which can be an early sign of cancer. Patients should engage actively in discussions about their biopsy results and what they mean for their ongoing management.

To facilitate tracking, patients should maintain a record of their endoscopic findings and any changes in their symptoms. This information can help guide future medical decisions and promote a collaborative approach to managing Barrett's Esophagus.

The Role of Proton Pump Inhibitors (PPIs)

Proton pump inhibitors (PPIs) play a significant role in managing Barrett's Esophagus by reducing stomach acid production. These medications help alleviate symptoms of gastroesophageal reflux disease (GERD), which is often associated with BE. Patients should work with their healthcare providers to determine the appropriate type and dosage of PPI for their specific needs.

It's important to take PPIs as prescribed and discuss any side effects or concerns with a healthcare provider. Regular evaluations may be necessary to assess the effectiveness of the treatment and make adjustments as needed to ensure optimal symptom control.

Long-Term Medication Management

Long-term medication management is essential for individuals with Barrett's Esophagus to effectively control symptoms and prevent disease progression. This may include ongoing use of PPIs or other medications tailored to the patient's specific symptoms and health status. Patients should have regular check-ins with their healthcare provider to monitor the effectiveness of their medication regimen.

Patients should also be aware of the importance of adherence to prescribed medications, as inconsistent use can lead to worsened symptoms and increased risks of complications. Engaging in open communication with healthcare providers can help ensure that any necessary adjustments are made promptly.

Lifestyle Measures to Prevent Progression

Incorporating lifestyle measures can significantly prevent the progression of Barrett's Esophagus. Patients should focus on maintaining a healthy weight through a balanced diet and regular exercise. Avoiding smoking and excessive alcohol consumption is also crucial, as these habits can exacerbate symptoms and increase the risk of complications.

Additionally, stress management techniques such as yoga, meditation, or deep breathing exercises can contribute to better overall health. Engaging in these lifestyle changes creates a supportive environment for esophageal health and empowers patients to take charge of their condition.

Avoiding Over-the-Counter Remedies without Advice

Individuals with Barrett's Esophagus should avoid using over-the-counter (OTC) remedies without first consulting their healthcare provider. Some OTC medications, while seemingly harmless, can interact negatively with prescribed treatments or exacerbate symptoms. Discussing all medications and supplements with a healthcare professional ensures safe and effective management.

Patients should also be cautious about relying on OTC solutions as a substitute for proper medical care. It's crucial to report any new symptoms or concerns to a healthcare provider to ensure comprehensive treatment and monitoring of Barrett's Esophagus.

Seeking Early Intervention for New Symptoms

Seeking early intervention for new symptoms is vital for individuals with Barrett's Esophagus to prevent complications. Patients should remain vigilant and promptly report any changes, such as increased difficulty swallowing, persistent heartburn, or unexplained weight loss. Early medical evaluation can lead to necessary diagnostic procedures and timely treatment.

Establishing a supportive relationship with healthcare providers can encourage patients to voice their concerns without hesitation. By prioritizing open communication, patients can significantly enhance their health management and outcomes related to Barrett's Esophagus.

Immunization Against Infections That May Affect Digestion

Immunization against infections that may affect digestion can be an important aspect of preventive care for those with Barrett's Esophagus. Patients should discuss vaccination options with their healthcare provider to ensure they are protected against infections like influenza and pneumococcal disease, which can impact overall health and complicate existing conditions.

Staying updated with vaccinations not only helps prevent illness but also supports a healthier digestive system. Patients should make it a routine practice to review their immunization history during check-ups to ensure they are adequately protected.

Being Proactive in Health Management

Being proactive in health management is crucial for individuals with Barrett's Esophagus. Patients should educate themselves about their condition, understand potential complications, and actively engage in their treatment plans. Setting health goals, maintaining regular medical appointments, and adhering to prescribed therapies are vital components of effective management.

Additionally, individuals should develop a support network, whether through family, friends, or support groups, to share experiences and gain insights. A proactive approach empowers patients to take control of their health and enhances their ability to navigate the challenges associated with Barrett's Esophagus.

CHAPTER 5:

Reducing Cancer Risk

Understanding the Risk of Esophageal Cancer in Barrett's Patients

Barrett's Esophagus significantly increases the risk of esophageal cancer, as the normal esophageal lining is replaced with abnormal cells due to chronic acid exposure. This condition can lead to dysplasia, where the cells become precancerous. Regular screening is essential for patients with Barrett's to monitor any changes in cell structure that could indicate progression to cancer.

To mitigate risk, patients should be aware of symptoms such as difficulty swallowing, persistent heartburn, or unexplained weight loss. Early detection through endoscopic surveillance can help identify dysplasia, allowing for timely intervention. It's crucial to maintain regular follow-up appointments with a healthcare provider for personalized risk assessments.

Role of Regular Monitoring in Cancer Prevention

Regular monitoring through endoscopy is vital for patients with Barrett's Esophagus, as it helps identify precancerous changes early. Healthcare professionals typically recommend surveillance every 1 to 3 years, depending on the degree of dysplasia. This allows for timely detection and treatment of any abnormal changes, thereby improving the chances of successful intervention.

During these monitoring sessions, biopsies may be performed to assess cell changes. Patients should discuss their individual monitoring schedule with their doctor and adhere to it strictly to maximize the effectiveness of cancer prevention strategies.

Lifestyle Changes to Reduce Cancer Risk

Implementing lifestyle changes can significantly lower the risk of esophageal cancer for those with Barrett's Esophagus. Key modifications include maintaining a healthy weight, engaging in regular physical activity, and reducing stress. These changes not only improve overall health but also enhance digestive function and lower acid reflux symptoms.

Additionally, it is essential to adopt habits such as eating smaller, more frequent meals and avoiding eating close to bedtime. These practical steps can help minimize acid exposure in the esophagus, thus reducing cancer risk.

Importance of Smoking Cessation

Quitting smoking is one of the most impactful lifestyle changes for individuals with Barrett's Esophagus. Smoking contributes to acid reflux and can accelerate the progression of Barrett's to esophageal cancer.

Support systems, such as counseling and nicotine replacement therapies, can aid in this process.

To successfully quit, patients should set a quit date and seek resources like support groups or hotlines that specialize in smoking cessation. Incorporating stress-relief techniques and engaging in physical activities can also help manage cravings and maintain motivation.

Managing Alcohol Consumption

Reducing alcohol intake is crucial for patients with Barrett's Esophagus, as alcohol can exacerbate acid reflux symptoms and irritate the esophagus. Patients are encouraged to limit their consumption to moderate levels or abstain altogether. Keeping a food and drink diary can help track intake and identify triggers.

Practical strategies include substituting alcoholic beverages with non-alcoholic options or setting specific limits on drinking occasions. Discussing personal goals with healthcare providers can also help reinforce the importance of moderation and support accountability.

Dietary Antioxidants for Esophageal Health

Incorporating dietary antioxidants can support esophageal health by combating oxidative stress and inflammation. Foods rich in antioxidants, such as berries, nuts, and green leafy vegetables, should be included in daily meals. A colorful plate can often indicate a variety of antioxidants and nutrients beneficial for the esophagus.

For practical implementation, patients can start by integrating a variety of fruits and vegetables into snacks and meals. Preparing smoothies or salads with antioxidant-rich ingredients can be a delicious and easy way to enhance diet quality.

Importance of Fiber-Rich Foods

A fiber-rich diet is essential for promoting digestive health and reducing cancer risk in Barrett's patients. Foods such as whole grains, legumes, fruits, and vegetables provide the necessary fiber to support healthy digestion and regular bowel movements. This can also help reduce acid reflux symptoms by improving gut health.

To increase fiber intake, patients can gradually incorporate high-fiber foods into their meals. Simple changes, like swapping white bread for whole grain or adding beans to salads, can make a significant difference without overwhelming the digestive system.

Benefits of Plant-Based Diets

Adopting a plant-based diet has been linked to lower cancer risk and improved digestive health. This diet emphasizes whole, minimally processed foods like fruits, vegetables, whole grains, and legumes, which can help reduce inflammation and provide essential nutrients. Patients with Barrett's are encouraged to explore plant-based meal options that align with their health goals.

To start transitioning, individuals can experiment with one meatless meal per week and explore new recipes centered around plant-based ingredients. Joining a local cooking class or online community can also provide inspiration and support in adopting this lifestyle.

Screening for Dysplasia (Pre-Cancerous Cells)

Screening for dysplasia is a critical component of care for patients with Barrett's Esophagus. Endoscopic procedures, such as esophagogastroduodenoscopy (EGD), allow doctors to visually inspect the esophagus and take biopsies of suspicious areas for laboratory analysis. These screenings are essential for detecting early precancerous changes.

Patients should discuss with their healthcare provider about the recommended frequency of screenings based on their individual risk factors. Staying informed about the process can alleviate anxiety and ensure that patients are prepared for their appointments.

Treatments for Dysplasia in Barrett's Patients

Treatment options for dysplasia in Barrett's Esophagus vary depending on the severity of the dysplastic changes. Options include endoscopic procedures such as radiofrequency ablation, which destroys abnormal cells while preserving healthy tissue. In more severe cases, esophagectomy (surgical removal of part or the entire esophagus) may be considered.

Patients should have open discussions with their healthcare team about the potential benefits and risks of each treatment option. Understanding the treatment process can empower patients and help them make informed decisions about their care.

Medications That Reduce Cancer Risk

Certain medications can help reduce cancer risk in patients with Barrett's Esophagus. Proton pump inhibitors (PPIs) are often prescribed to manage acid reflux, and they may also lower the risk of progression to cancer. Regular follow-up with a healthcare provider is necessary to ensure the appropriate medication is being used and to monitor any side effects.

Patients should adhere to their prescribed medication regimen and discuss any concerns or side effects with their doctor. Staying engaged in their treatment plan is vital for optimizing their esophageal health.

Role of Surgical Interventions in High-Risk Cases

For patients identified as high-risk for esophageal cancer, surgical interventions may be necessary to manage Barrett's Esophagus effectively. Surgical options include esophagectomy or endoscopic resection of dysplastic lesions. These procedures can help remove cancerous or precancerous tissues, significantly lowering cancer risk.

Patients should engage in thorough discussions with their healthcare providers about the surgical options available, including potential benefits and recovery processes. Understanding what to expect can help ease anxiety and prepare individuals for the necessary lifestyle adjustments post-surgery.

Importance of Early Detection in Cancer Prevention

Early detection of Barrett's Esophagus and its potential progression to cancer is crucial for successful outcomes. Regular screenings and awareness of symptoms can lead to timely intervention, drastically improving prognosis. Patients should stay vigilant for changes in their health and maintain open communication with their healthcare providers.

Establishing a personalized monitoring plan and adhering to it can significantly impact long-term health outcomes. By prioritizing regular check-ups and symptom awareness, patients can take proactive steps toward preventing esophageal cancer.

CHAPTER 6:

Dietary Changes for Esophageal Health

Foods to Avoid for Barrett's Esophagus

Individuals with Barrett's esophagus should avoid foods that can trigger or exacerbate gastroesophageal reflux disease (GERD) symptoms. Common culprits include spicy foods, chocolate, caffeinated beverages, carbonated drinks, and high-fat foods. These items can relax the lower esophageal sphincter, allowing stomach acid to rise into the esophagus and potentially worsen inflammation and irritation.

In addition to these, acidic foods such as citrus fruits, tomatoes, and vinegar should be limited, as they can further irritate the esophagus. Processed foods high in sugar and unhealthy fats should also be avoided, as they can promote inflammation. Keeping a food diary to track reactions can help identify specific foods that may worsen symptoms, leading to more personalized dietary choices.

Best Foods for Soothing the Esophagus

Soothing foods can play a significant role in managing Barrett's esophagus symptoms. Options like oatmeal, whole grain bread, and bananas are gentle on the digestive system and can help coat the esophagus. Incorporating lean proteins, such as chicken, turkey, and fish, is also beneficial, as they are less likely to trigger reflux compared to fried or fatty meats.

In addition, yogurt and other probiotic-rich foods can support gut health and aid digestion. These foods can help mitigate symptoms and provide essential nutrients. When preparing meals, consider incorporating foods that are moist and easy to swallow to minimize discomfort.

Importance of a Balanced, Anti-Inflammatory Diet

A balanced, anti-inflammatory diet is crucial for individuals with Barrett's esophagus, as it can help reduce inflammation and support overall digestive health. This diet should emphasize whole foods such as fruits, vegetables, whole grains, and lean proteins while minimizing processed and refined foods. Foods rich in omega-3 fatty acids, like salmon and walnuts, can help combat inflammation.

To create an anti-inflammatory meal plan, consider including a variety of colorful fruits and vegetables, as they contain antioxidants that promote healing. Planning meals around whole foods and reducing reliance on convenience foods will foster a healthier gut environment and contribute to better digestive health.

How Fatty Foods Exacerbate Reflux

Fatty foods can exacerbate GERD symptoms by relaxing the lower esophageal sphincter (LES), which allows stomach acid to flow back into the esophagus. Foods high in saturated and trans fats, such as fried foods, fatty cuts of meat, and certain dairy products, should be limited or avoided. These foods not only worsen reflux symptoms but can also contribute to weight gain, which can further increase reflux episodes.

To mitigate these effects, focus on healthier fat sources like avocados, nuts, and olive oil, which are less likely to provoke symptoms. Preparing meals using cooking methods such as grilling, baking, or steaming instead of frying can help reduce the fat content and promote esophageal health.

Benefits of Whole Grains for Digestion

Whole grains are an excellent choice for individuals with Barrett's esophagus as they are rich in fiber, which aids digestion and helps maintain regular bowel movements. Foods like brown rice, quinoa, whole grain bread, and oats can help prevent constipation and promote a healthy gut environment. Additionally, fiber can help absorb excess stomach acid, further reducing the risk of irritation.

To incorporate more whole grains into your diet, replace refined grains with whole grain alternatives. For example, choose whole grain pasta instead of regular pasta and opt for brown rice instead of white rice. Gradually increasing fiber intake can also help your digestive system adjust without discomfort.

The Role of Fruits and Vegetables in Esophageal Health

Fruits and vegetables are vital for esophageal health due to their high antioxidant content and ability to provide essential vitamins and minerals. They can help combat inflammation and promote healing in the esophagus. Including a variety of colorful fruits and vegetables in your daily diet ensures a wide range of nutrients that can benefit your overall health.

In practical terms, aim for at least five servings of fruits and vegetables each day. Smoothies can be a great way to combine various fruits and vegetables for a nutrient-packed meal or snack. Cooking methods such as steaming or baking can enhance the palatability of these foods while retaining their nutritional value.

Avoiding Acidic Foods and Beverages

Acidic foods and beverages can irritate the esophagus and worsen symptoms for those with Barrett's esophagus. It is advisable to limit or avoid citrus fruits, tomatoes, coffee, alcohol, and carbonated drinks. These items can trigger heartburn and discomfort by increasing acidity in the stomach.

To minimize acid intake, consider substituting acidic beverages with herbal teas or water infused with non-citrus fruits. When consuming foods like tomatoes, opt for low-acid varieties or cook them to reduce their acidity. Keeping track of how your body responds to certain foods can guide you in making better dietary choices.

How to Identify Personal Food Triggers

Identifying personal food triggers is an essential step in managing Barrett's esophagus. Keeping a food diary can help track what you eat and how it affects your symptoms. Note any meals or snacks that lead to discomfort, allowing you to pinpoint specific foods or ingredients to avoid in the future.

Experiment with elimination diets, where you remove suspected trigger foods for a few weeks and gradually reintroduce them one at a time. This method can help you understand how different foods impact your esophageal health and enable you to create a personalized, symptom-friendly diet.

Importance of Regular, Smaller Meals

Eating regular, smaller meals can help manage Barrett's esophagus by preventing excessive stomach distension, which can lead to reflux. Instead of three large meals a day, aim for five to six smaller meals to keep stomach pressure low and reduce the likelihood of acid reflux. This approach can also help regulate blood sugar levels and provide a steady source of energy throughout the day.

When planning your meals, consider portion sizes and avoid overloading your plate. Prepping meals in advance can help you stick to this routine and make it easier to avoid large portions during mealtimes. Also, be mindful of eating slowly and chewing your food thoroughly to aid digestion.

Hydration: How Much Water is Beneficial?

Staying hydrated is crucial for digestive health, particularly for individuals with Barrett's esophagus. Drinking enough water helps dilute stomach acid and supports overall digestive function. Aim for at least eight 8-ounce glasses of water a day, adjusting based on your activity level and climate.

To encourage hydration, keep a water bottle handy throughout the day and set reminders to drink regularly. Herbal teas can also be a soothing alternative to plain water, providing hydration without irritating the esophagus. Avoid drinking large amounts of water during meals, as it can increase stomach pressure.

Preparing Easy, Reflux-Friendly Recipes

Preparing reflux-friendly recipes can make managing Barrett's esophagus more enjoyable and less restrictive. Focus on using gentle cooking methods such as steaming, baking, or grilling to keep meals light and healthy. Incorporate ingredients that are easy on the stomach, like lean proteins, whole grains, and plenty of fruits and vegetables.

Simple recipes like baked chicken with steamed broccoli and quinoa or oatmeal with bananas and honey can provide nutritious meals without triggering symptoms. Experiment with different herbs and spices to add flavor without the heat that can exacerbate reflux. Meal prepping can also save time and ensure you have healthy options readily available.

Use of Herbs and Spices for Digestion

Herbs and spices can enhance flavor while promoting digestive health, making them a great addition to meals for those with Barrett's esophagus. Gentle options like ginger, turmeric, and peppermint have anti-inflammatory properties and can aid in digestion. Incorporating these into your meals can help alleviate discomfort and promote better gut health.

When using herbs and spices, start with small amounts to see how your body responds. Fresh herbs like basil, parsley, and dill can add flavor without the risk of reflux. Consider using herbal teas or adding spices to dishes that are known for their soothing qualities to enhance overall well-being.

Seeking Advice from a Nutritionist

Consulting with a nutritionist can provide valuable guidance for managing Barrett's esophagus and optimizing your diet. A qualified nutritionist can help assess your specific dietary needs, identify potential food triggers, and create a personalized meal plan that supports digestive health. They can also provide insight into proper portion sizes and meal timing to minimize reflux symptoms.

To find a nutritionist, look for a registered dietitian with experience in gastrointestinal health. Many nutritionists offer virtual consultations, making it easier to access their expertise. Collaborating with a professional can empower you to make informed dietary choices and improve your overall quality of life.

CHAPTER 7:

Medical Treatments for Barrett's Esophagus

Common Medications Prescribed for Barrett's

Barrett's esophagus often requires medication to manage symptoms and prevent progression. Commonly prescribed medications include proton pump inhibitors (PPIs), H2 blockers, and occasionally, medications to control acid reflux. Patients should always consult their healthcare provider to determine the most appropriate medication based on individual symptoms and health conditions.

When taking these medications, it's essential to follow the prescribed dosage and frequency. Regular follow-ups with your healthcare provider can help assess the effectiveness of the treatment and make necessary adjustments to the medication regimen. Keeping a symptom diary can also aid in discussing medication efficacy during appointments.

Role of Proton Pump Inhibitors (PPIs)

Proton pump inhibitors (PPIs) play a crucial role in managing Barrett's esophagus by reducing stomach acid production, which helps alleviate symptoms of gastroesophageal reflux disease (GERD). By lowering acid levels, PPIs can promote healing of the esophagus and reduce inflammation. They are often prescribed for long-term use in patients with Barrett's to help prevent further damage to the esophagus.

To use PPIs effectively, take them 30 to 60 minutes before meals, usually once daily. It's essential to follow your healthcare provider's instructions regarding dosage and duration of therapy, as improper use can lead to decreased effectiveness. Monitoring symptoms and side effects is vital to ensure the medication is working as intended.

Understanding H2 Blockers

H2 blockers are another class of medications used to treat Barrett's esophagus by reducing the amount of acid produced by the stomach. Unlike PPIs, H2 blockers can provide quicker relief from heartburn and acid reflux symptoms, making them a good option for occasional use or in combination with PPIs. Common H2 blockers include ranitidine and famotidine.

To use H2 blockers effectively, take them as directed, typically about an hour before meals. If symptoms persist despite medication, consult your healthcare provider for potential adjustments in treatment or additional therapies that may be more suitable.

Over-the-Counter Antacid Usage

Over-the-counter antacids can provide quick relief from heartburn and indigestion for individuals with Barrett's esophagus. These medications neutralize stomach acid and can be taken as needed, often within a few hours of meals or when symptoms arise. Popular antacids include calcium carbonate (Tums) and magnesium hydroxide (Maalox).

To maximize the benefits of antacids, it's important to read the instructions carefully regarding dosage and frequency. However, relying solely on antacids may not address the underlying issues associated with Barrett's, so it is advisable to consult a healthcare provider for a comprehensive treatment plan.

Endoscopic Therapies to Treat Barrett's

Endoscopic therapies are minimally invasive procedures used to treat Barrett's esophagus, particularly in patients with dysplasia (pre-cancerous changes). Common endoscopic treatments include radiofrequency ablation (RFA) and photodynamic therapy (PDT), which aim to remove or destroy abnormal cells in the esophagus. These procedures are typically performed in specialized clinics or hospitals.

Preparation for endoscopic therapy may involve fasting for several hours prior to the procedure. Patients should discuss any medications they are taking with their healthcare provider, as some may need to be paused temporarily. Post-procedure care usually includes monitoring for any side effects and follow-up appointments to evaluate the effectiveness of the treatment.

Radiofrequency Ablation (RFA) Explained

Radiofrequency ablation (RFA) is a specific type of endoscopic therapy that uses heat generated by radio waves to destroy abnormal cells in the esophagus. RFA is often recommended for patients with high-grade dysplasia and aims to reduce the risk of esophageal cancer. The procedure is typically outpatient, and recovery is usually quick.

During RFA, the patient is sedated, and a special device is inserted into the esophagus to deliver the radiofrequency energy. Post-procedure, patients may experience some discomfort or difficulty swallowing, which usually resolves within a few days. Regular follow-up appointments are crucial to monitor the esophagus and ensure successful treatment.

Photodynamic Therapy (PDT) for Dysplasia

Photodynamic therapy (PDT) is another endoscopic treatment option for Barrett's esophagus with dysplasia. This therapy involves administering a light-sensitive medication that accumulates in abnormal cells. After a waiting period, a specific wavelength of light is used to activate the medication, destroying the targeted cells.

Patients typically require a few hours of preparation before the procedure, including avoiding certain medications. After PDT, some swelling and discomfort may occur, but these effects generally diminish within a few days. Regular follow-up care is essential to assess the response to treatment and to detect any recurrence of dysplasia.

Cryotherapy: What to Expect

Cryotherapy is an emerging treatment for Barrett's esophagus that involves freezing abnormal cells in the esophagus. This procedure is performed using a cryoballoon or spray, which applies extremely cold temperatures to destroy the targeted tissue. Cryotherapy can be an effective option for patients with dysplasia who have not responded to other treatments.

Before undergoing cryotherapy, patients may need to fast and stop certain medications. The procedure is typically done under sedation, and recovery may involve some soreness in the throat and difficulty swallowing. Follow-up appointments are critical to monitor healing and check for any signs of dysplasia.

When Surgery is recommended

Surgery for Barrett's esophagus is typically considered when other treatments have failed or in cases of high-grade dysplasia. The most common surgical procedure is esophagectomy, which involves removing the affected portion of the esophagus. This option may be necessary for patients at high risk for esophageal cancer.

Patients considering surgery should discuss the risks and benefits with their healthcare provider, including potential complications and recovery time. Preoperative assessments may involve imaging studies and consultations with specialists. Post-surgery, patients will require a structured recovery plan, including dietary modifications and regular follow-up visits.

Medications for Acid Suppression

In addition to PPIs and H2 blockers, other medications for acid suppression may be used in managing Barrett's esophagus. These can include prokinetic agents that help improve esophageal motility and reduce reflux symptoms. Understanding the specific medication and its purpose can enhance adherence and symptom management.

It's essential to take these medications as directed and to have open communication with healthcare providers regarding any side effects or concerns. Regular monitoring of symptoms can help determine the effectiveness of the treatment and inform future adjustments to the medication plan.

How Long to Continue Medication Therapy

The duration of medication therapy for Barrett's esophagus varies based on individual patient needs and response to treatment. Generally, PPIs may be recommended for long-term use to manage symptoms and prevent progression, while H2 blockers may be used for shorter durations. Regular follow-ups with a healthcare provider are crucial to assess the need for ongoing therapy.

Patients should not stop or adjust their medications without consulting their healthcare provider. If symptoms improve, doctors may consider tapering medications to find the lowest effective dose. Ongoing monitoring and assessment can help guide the decision-making process regarding medication duration.

Pros and Cons of Long-Term Medication Use

Long-term medication use for Barrett's esophagus has both advantages and disadvantages. On the positive side, medications such as PPIs effectively reduce acid production, alleviate symptoms, and decrease the risk of esophageal damage. Consistent use can improve the quality of life for many patients.

However, long-term medication can also come with drawbacks, including potential side effects like nutrient malabsorption, kidney issues, and increased risk of certain infections. Patients should engage in discussions with their healthcare provider about the risks and benefits of long-term therapy, as well as explore non-pharmacological strategies to manage symptoms.

Potential Side Effects of Common Treatments

Like any medical treatments, therapies for Barrett's esophagus may have potential side effects. Common medications such as PPIs can lead to headaches, gastrointestinal issues, and increased susceptibility to infections. Endoscopic therapies may result in throat discomfort, difficulty swallowing, or bleeding, although serious complications are rare.

Patients should be vigilant in reporting any unusual symptoms or side effects to their healthcare provider. Ongoing communication can help manage side effects effectively and may prompt adjustments in the treatment plan to optimize patient comfort and care.

CHAPTER 8:

Surgical Options and Interventions

When Surgery Becomes Necessary

Surgery for Barrett's esophagus is often considered when there are severe dysplastic changes in the esophagus or when symptoms are unmanageable despite optimal medical therapy. If routine monitoring shows worsening conditions or if there's a significant risk of progression to esophageal cancer, surgical options may become necessary. A gastroenterologist will evaluate your symptoms, perform endoscopies, and determine the best surgical approach based on the severity of the changes.

Before undergoing surgery, discuss your overall health and any other conditions with your healthcare provider. They will guide you through the decision-making process, weighing the benefits against the risks. It's essential to understand the type of surgery recommended, the expected outcomes, and any lifestyle changes required post-surgery.

Nissen Fundoplication: GERD Surgery

Nissen fundoplication is a common surgical procedure used to treat gastroesophageal reflux disease (GERD), especially when lifestyle changes and medications are insufficient. During this procedure, the top of the stomach is wrapped around the lower esophagus to reinforce the lower esophageal sphincter, preventing acid reflux. Patients typically receive general anesthesia, and the surgery can be done through traditional or minimally invasive techniques.

Post-surgery, many patients report significant relief from GERD symptoms, such as heartburn and regurgitation. Recovery involves following a specific diet and gradually reintroducing foods. Patients should work closely with their healthcare providers to ensure successful outcomes and manage any complications that may arise.

Understanding Esophagectomy (Esophagus Removal)

Esophagectomy is a surgical procedure that involves the removal of part or all of the esophagus, often due to severe dysplasia or esophageal cancer. This procedure can significantly impact a patient's ability to swallow and digest food, as a new connection must be established between the stomach and the remaining esophagus or throat. Pre-operative assessments, including imaging and endoscopy, will help determine the extent of the surgery required.

After esophagectomy, patients often face a challenging recovery period. They may need to adapt to a new diet, which often starts with liquid foods and gradually progresses to more solid options. Regular follow-ups with healthcare providers are crucial to monitor healing and adjust dietary needs accordingly.

Recovery Expectations Post-Surgery

Recovery from esophageal surgery can vary significantly based on the type of procedure performed and the individual's overall health. Patients should expect a hospital stay ranging from a few days to a week, depending on the complexity of the surgery. Pain management, respiratory exercises, and mobility will be emphasized during this time to enhance recovery.

At home, recovery can take several weeks to months. It is essential to gradually increase physical activity and adhere to dietary guidelines provided by healthcare professionals. Monitoring for signs of complications, such as infection or difficulty swallowing, are crucial, and patients should maintain open communication with their healthcare team throughout their recovery journey.

Minimally Invasive Surgery Options

Minimally invasive surgery for Barrett's esophagus or GERD, such as laparoscopic techniques, involves smaller incisions, resulting in less pain, reduced recovery time, and shorter hospital stays. Surgeons may use tools like endoscopes and robotic assistance to perform procedures with greater precision. Patients should consult with their surgeons about the feasibility of minimally invasive options based on their specific medical conditions.

Candidates for minimally invasive surgery typically undergo extensive pre-operative assessments to ensure they are suitable for this type of intervention. The recovery process is generally quicker than traditional surgery, allowing patients to return to normal activities sooner while still requiring careful monitoring for any post-operative complications.

Risks Associated with Surgical Interventions

Surgical interventions for Barrett's esophagus come with inherent risks, including infection, bleeding, and complications related to anesthesia. Specific to esophageal surgeries, patients may experience difficulty swallowing, reflux, or changes in bowel habits. It's important to have a thorough discussion with your surgeon about these risks prior to surgery, including their likelihood and how they can be managed.

In addition to immediate risks, patients should be aware of long-term complications such as strictures or changes in esophageal motility. Maintaining open communication with healthcare providers during the recovery phase will facilitate the early detection of any adverse effects and allow for timely intervention.

Post-Surgery Diet and Care

After esophageal surgery, patients must adhere to a specific diet to aid in recovery and ensure the proper healing of the surgical site. Initially, a liquid diet is recommended, progressing to soft foods before gradually reintroducing solid foods. It's vital to eat smaller, more frequent meals and chew food thoroughly to ease digestion.

Healthcare providers may recommend nutritional supplements to ensure adequate calorie and protein intake during the recovery phase. Monitoring for symptoms such as pain, nausea, or difficulty swallowing is essential, and any concerns should be promptly discussed with a healthcare professional for appropriate management.

Importance of Follow-Up After Surgery

Regular follow-up appointments after esophageal surgery are crucial for monitoring recovery and addressing any complications that may arise. Healthcare providers will assess healing, manage symptoms, and perform necessary diagnostic tests, such as endoscopies, to ensure there are no signs of cancer recurrence or other issues.

Patients should be proactive in attending these appointments and communicating any new or worsening symptoms. A solid follow-up plan will help ensure long-term success and quality of life post-surgery.

Surgical Alternatives to Managing Reflux

For patients who are not suitable candidates for surgery or prefer to avoid it, several non-surgical alternatives can effectively manage reflux symptoms. These include lifestyle changes such as weight loss, dietary modifications, and medication management with proton pump inhibitors (PPIs) or H2 blockers. Discussing these options with a healthcare provider can help tailor a plan suited to individual needs.

Some newer procedures, such as endoscopic therapies, offer alternatives to traditional surgery. These methods can provide symptom relief without the need for more invasive surgery, making them appealing for those seeking less drastic measures while still addressing their reflux issues.

When to Opt for Non-Surgical Treatments

Non-surgical treatments should be considered when symptoms are mild or manageable and when patients prefer to explore lifestyle changes or medications before considering surgical options. Patients experiencing occasional heartburn may find relief through over-the-counter medications, while those with more persistent symptoms might require prescription treatments or lifestyle adjustments.

If medications and lifestyle changes fail to provide adequate relief, it may be time to discuss surgical options with a healthcare provider. Understanding the severity of symptoms and how they affect daily life will guide the decision-making process regarding the best treatment approach.

Palliative Care for Late-Stage Esophageal Cancer

Palliative care focuses on providing relief from the symptoms and stress of late-stage esophageal cancer, aiming to enhance the quality of life for patients and their families. This approach can involve pain management, nutritional support, and psychological care, addressing both physical and emotional needs. Patients should discuss palliative options with their healthcare team to understand how these services can support their overall well-being.

Involving a multidisciplinary team, including oncologists, nurses, social workers, and nutritionists, can create a comprehensive care plan. This collaboration ensures that all aspects of a patient's health and comfort are addressed, making the experience more manageable during this challenging time.

Seeking Second Opinions Before Surgery

Obtaining a second opinion before proceeding with surgery is a prudent step for anyone facing major medical decisions. Consulting another specialist can provide additional insights, confirm diagnoses, and present alternative treatment options. Patients should feel empowered to seek second opinions to ensure they fully understand their condition and treatment options.

When seeking a second opinion, patients should provide the new physician with all relevant medical records and imaging results. Open communication about any concerns or questions regarding the recommended surgery will help facilitate a thorough evaluation and informed decision-making.

How to Choose a Specialist Surgeon

Choosing a specialist surgeon for esophageal conditions is crucial for achieving the best outcomes. Patients should look for surgeons who are board-certified in general surgery and have specific experience in esophageal procedures. Researching their credentials, success rates, and patient reviews can provide insight into their expertise and approach to care.

It's also important to consider the surgeon's communication style and whether you feel comfortable discussing your concerns with them. A collaborative relationship will facilitate better care and ensure that you are well-informed throughout the surgical process.

CHAPTER 9:

Common Concerns and FAQs

Can Barrett's Esophagus be reversed?

While Barrett's Esophagus itself cannot be completely reversed, its progression can be managed effectively. The primary focus should be on controlling gastroesophageal reflux disease (GERD) symptoms, as reducing acid exposure can help minimize damage to the esophagus. This may involve a combination of lifestyle changes, dietary adjustments, and medications to lower acid production and promote healing.

In some cases, medical interventions such as endoscopic procedures may be recommended to remove abnormal cells or promote healing. Regular follow-up with your healthcare provider is essential for monitoring your condition and adapting your treatment plan as needed to optimize esophageal health.

What are the chances of developing cancer?

Individuals with Barrett's Esophagus are at a higher risk of developing esophageal cancer compared to the general population, but the risk is still relatively low. Studies suggest that approximately 0.5% to 1% of patients with Barrett's Esophagus will develop esophageal adenocarcinoma each year. Regular monitoring through endoscopic screenings helps identify any dysplastic changes early, allowing for timely intervention.

It's important to remember that not everyone with Barrett's will develop cancer. The risk factors include the extent of dysplasia, duration of Barrett's Esophagus, and lifestyle factors such as smoking and obesity. Discussing personal risk factors with your healthcare provider can provide a clearer understanding of your specific situation.

How often should I get screened?

Screening frequency for Barrett's Esophagus typically depends on the degree of dysplasia present. If no dysplasia is found, follow-up endoscopies may be recommended every three to five years. However, if low-grade dysplasia is detected, your doctor might suggest annual screenings to monitor for progression. High-grade dysplasia may require more immediate attention and treatment options.

It's crucial to maintain open communication with your healthcare provider regarding your specific screening schedule. Adhering to recommended screening intervals can lead to early detection and treatment of any changes that could indicate cancer progression.

Will I need lifelong medication?

Many individuals with Barrett's Esophagus will require lifelong medication, particularly proton pump inhibitors (PPIs), to control acid reflux symptoms. These medications reduce stomach acid production, helping to alleviate symptoms and protect the esophagus from further damage. Your doctor will determine the most appropriate medication and dosage for your condition.

However, medication alone may not suffice. A comprehensive approach that includes lifestyle changes, dietary modifications, and regular monitoring is essential for managing Barrett's Esophagus effectively. Always consult your healthcare provider before making any changes to your medication regimen.

What foods should I avoid permanently?

To manage Barrett's Esophagus effectively, certain foods should be avoided to minimize acid reflux and irritation. Common culprits include spicy foods, acidic items (like citrus fruits and tomatoes), caffeine, chocolate, and fatty or fried foods. Identifying and eliminating personal triggers through a food diary can help tailor dietary choices to your specific needs.

In addition to avoiding certain foods, incorporating a diet rich in fruits, vegetables, whole grains, and lean proteins can promote overall digestive health. Staying hydrated and opting for smaller, more frequent meals instead of large portions can also alleviate symptoms and reduce discomfort.

How can I reduce nighttime symptoms?

To minimize nighttime symptoms of Barrett's Esophagus, consider adjusting your sleeping position by elevating the head of your bed by 6 to 8 inches. This elevation helps prevent stomach acid from flowing back into the esophagus during sleep. Additionally, avoid eating large meals or snacking close to bedtime, as this can trigger nighttime reflux.

Establishing a calming bedtime routine, including avoiding stimulants and practicing relaxation techniques, can further reduce symptoms. Over-the-counter antacids may provide temporary relief, but consult your healthcare provider for more effective long-term solutions tailored to your condition.

Is it safe to exercise with Barrett's Esophagus?

Exercise is generally safe for individuals with Barrett's Esophagus and can contribute positively to overall health. Engaging in moderate physical activity can help maintain a healthy weight, which is crucial for reducing reflux symptoms. Activities like walking, swimming, or yoga can be beneficial; however, avoid high-impact exercises that may exacerbate symptoms.

Listening to your body is key; if certain activities cause discomfort, consider modifying them or choosing gentler alternatives. Staying hydrated and avoiding exercising right after meals can also help manage symptoms effectively during physical activity.

Can stress make my condition worse?

Stress can play a significant role in exacerbating symptoms of Barrett's Esophagus and GERD. Increased stress levels may lead to heightened acid production and muscle tension, contributing to discomfort. Incorporating stress management techniques such as deep breathing, meditation, or yoga can help alleviate symptoms and promote overall well-being.

Engaging in regular physical activity and maintaining a balanced diet can also serve as effective stress relievers. Consider reaching out for support from friends, family, or a mental health professional to help manage stress effectively and improve your digestive health.

What are the signs that Barrett's is progressing?

Signs that Barrett's Esophagus may be progressing include worsening symptoms of gastroesophageal reflux, such as increased heartburn, regurgitation, difficulty swallowing, or chest pain. If you notice these changes or experience new symptoms like weight loss or persistent nausea, it's essential to consult your healthcare provider promptly for evaluation.

Regular surveillance through endoscopic procedures is critical for monitoring the condition and identifying any dysplastic changes early. Early intervention is key to preventing progression to esophageal cancer, so being vigilant about symptom changes and follow-up appointments is crucial.

Should I consider alternative therapies?

Alternative therapies can be considered as complementary approaches to managing Barrett's Esophagus. Options such as acupuncture, herbal remedies, and nutritional supplements may offer some relief from symptoms. However, it's essential to discuss these with your healthcare provider to ensure they are safe and do not interfere with prescribed treatments.

Research is still ongoing regarding the effectiveness of alternative therapies, so keeping an open dialogue with your healthcare team can help tailor a holistic approach that includes both conventional and alternative treatments. Monitoring your response to these therapies is crucial for determining their efficacy.

How do I talk to my family about my condition?

When discussing Barrett's Esophagus with family, it's helpful to approach the conversation with clarity and openness. Explain what the condition is, its symptoms, and how it affects your daily life. Providing educational resources can also help family members better understand your experience and offer their support.

Encouraging questions and expressing your feelings about the condition can foster a supportive environment. Involving family members in discussions about treatment options and lifestyle changes can also help them understand how they can assist you in managing your condition effectively.

Can lifestyle changes stop the progression of Barrett's?

Lifestyle changes play a crucial role in managing Barrett's Esophagus and may help prevent its progression. Adopting a healthy diet, maintaining a healthy weight, quitting smoking, and reducing alcohol intake can significantly lower the risk of worsening symptoms and associated complications.

Regular exercise, stress management techniques, and adhering to prescribed medications are also vital components of a comprehensive approach. While lifestyle changes may not completely reverse Barrett's, they can significantly improve your quality of life and lower cancer risk.

What is the latest research on Barrett's and esophageal cancer?

Recent research on Barrett's Esophagus and its association with esophageal cancer focuses on early detection methods, risk stratification, and potential treatments. Studies are exploring the role of biomarkers and genetic profiling to identify patients at higher risk for cancer development, which could lead to more tailored surveillance strategies.

Innovative treatments, such as radiofrequency ablation and endoscopic mucosal resection, are being investigated for their efficacy in removing dysplastic cells and reducing cancer risk. Staying informed about these developments through regular consultations with your healthcare provider can help you understand your options and make informed decisions about your health.

Conclusion

Summarizing the Importance of Early Detection and Ongoing Care

Early detection of Barrett's Esophagus is crucial because it allows for timely interventions that can prevent the progression to esophageal cancer. Regular screenings, such as endoscopies, enable healthcare providers to monitor changes in the esophagus and identify precancerous cells. The earlier these changes are detected, the more effective treatment options become, which can significantly reduce the risk of cancer.

Ongoing care is equally important, as Barrett's Esophagus requires continuous monitoring and management to ensure that the condition does not worsen. Patients should establish a regular follow-up schedule with their healthcare providers to assess symptoms, undergo necessary tests, and adjust treatment plans. This proactive approach helps maintain esophageal health and allows for prompt action if complications arise.

How Lifestyle and Medical Treatments Can Manage Barrett's Esophagus

Managing Barrett's Esophagus often involves a combination of lifestyle changes and medical treatments. Patients should focus on dietary modifications, such as avoiding spicy, acidic, and fatty foods, which can exacerbate symptoms. Incorporating smaller, more frequent meals can also help reduce reflux. Additionally, medications like proton pump inhibitors (PPIs) may be prescribed to lower stomach acid production, alleviating irritation in the esophagus.

In some cases, more invasive treatments may be necessary. Procedures like radiofrequency ablation or endoscopic mucosal resection can be performed to remove abnormal cells or tissue. It's essential for patients to work closely with their healthcare team to determine the most appropriate treatment options based on their individual health status and the severity of their condition.

Encouraging Regular Medical Check-ups and Monitoring

Regular medical check-ups are vital for individuals with Barrett's Esophagus, as they facilitate timely assessments of the condition. Patients should schedule follow-up appointments at least once a year, or more frequently as recommended by their healthcare provider. These check-ups often include endoscopic examinations to evaluate the esophagus and ensure any changes are detected early.

Monitoring involves not just physical examinations, but also staying alert to symptoms such as difficulty swallowing, chest pain, or unintentional weight loss. Patients should keep a symptom diary to share with their doctors, providing essential information that can guide treatment decisions and adjustments.

The Power of Dietary and Lifestyle Changes for Long-Term Health

Dietary and lifestyle changes play a significant role in managing Barrett's Esophagus and promoting long-term health. Patients are encouraged to adopt a Mediterranean-style diet rich in fruits, vegetables, whole grains, and lean proteins while minimizing processed foods and sugars. Maintaining a healthy weight through regular exercise and balanced nutrition can help reduce symptoms and lower the risk of disease progression.

Other lifestyle modifications include quitting smoking, reducing alcohol consumption, and elevating the head of the bed to prevent nighttime reflux. These changes can greatly enhance overall well-being and significantly improve the quality of life for individuals living with Barrett's Esophagus.

Importance of a Proactive, Informed Approach to Managing Barrett's

A proactive approach to managing Barrett's Esophagus is essential for optimizing health outcomes. Patients should educate themselves about their condition, including potential risks and symptoms to watch for. Being informed empowers individuals to take an active role in their care, facilitating better communication with healthcare providers and ensuring that they receive appropriate screenings and treatments.

Staying engaged in one's health journey also involves seeking out reliable information and support networks. Joining support groups or forums can provide encouragement and share experiences that help in coping with the challenges of living with Barrett's Esophagus, fostering a community of individuals who understand the importance of proactive management.

www.ingramcontent.com/pod-product-compliance
Lightning Source LLC
Chambersburg PA
CBHW071028250726
48653CB00005B/1765